Email : dani@danidfitness.com

For more information, visit our website at danidfitness.com

Disclaimer: This book is for informational purposes only and is intended to help guide you on your journey to a healthier life through movement. Dani D. Fitness is not a licensed therapist; she is a holistic health coach with 12 years of experience as a certified group fitness instructor and personal trainer. She has also run a successful business since 2017 and has gone through this journey just like you. This book is meant to be a tool and a starting point, not the ultimate solution for your relationship with your body and mind. The hope and goal are that you will start loving yourself more each day.

Table of Contents

Intro: Who is Dani D., owner of Dani D. Fitness

The Love Your Body Initiative

Chapter 1: What do you love about your body

Chapter 2: Why don't you love your body

Chapter 3: When did you start disliking your body

Chapter 4: Where are you in your journey of loving your body

Chapter 5: How to stay on your journey of loving your body throughout

People of all ages, sizes, and walks of life unite in believing in this mission. Here's what they have to say:

Intro: Who is Dani D., owner of Dani D. Fitness?

Dani D., short for Danielle Dyer, is a 31-year-old female entrepreneur from Murfreesboro, Tennessee. Dani grew up dancing from the age of 3 and competed in dance from the age of 10 to 18. Movement has always been a passion of hers. She now lives in Nashville, Tennessee, where she runs her business, Dani D. Fitness LLC, and produces her podcast, "The Love Your Body Podcast." She also has her own supplement called Fight Energy, created a dance fitness format, MoveFit that she has led thousands in over the last decade and was Nashville's Strongest Woman in 2019 for flipping a 500lb tire at a Strongman Competition!

She trains people all over the U.S. through her online programming and virtual training and has followers from all over the world. Growing up, Dani didn't have the typical body size for a dancer, let alone the "average" girl. She was always taller, had bigger feet, and had a broader build. She dealt with body shaming and verbal abuse, which led to body dysmorphia and unhealthy eating habits. After trying every diet growing up, she finally decided at age 19 that she wasn't doing this for anyone else anymore—she wanted to get healthy for herself. She knew she would never please everyone and felt trapped in a box that she needed to escape. Finally, she did, and she started learning how to eat for her body and goals and became a certified group fitness instructor, creating her own format, MoveFit. From there, she became a certified personal trainer, sports nutritionist, holistic health coach, strength training specialist and more throughout her career and even became an assistant helping with certifications to Master Trainer Susie Gorman Green through AAAI. After college she went to Vermont for a Fitness Internship at an all women's healthy lifestyle resort meeting women from all walks of life and learned everything she could about movement, fuel, recovery, and so much more while studying under an amazing mentor Lynn Ann Covell. While there she met a business mentor and now dear friend Claire Craven and learned that the dreams she always spoke of about making a difference in the world, could very much come true.

Doesn't mean that along the path especially when she started out it became very difficult to be taken seriously. She was always an outlier, even up until as recently as a few years ago. Because of how she felt growing up, she never wanted anyone to feel as alone as she did on her journey, and wanted to help as many as she could so she started her business on August 1, 2017. Now, she gets to support and help others feel empowered and strong throughout their journey and help them change the mindset that they too can break out of the box they've been placed in.

She wants you to know that no matter where you are on your journey, what's happened to you, or if you feel like you've tried everything, there is hope—and that hope is Dani D. Fitness LYB Method and Initiative. Read below for more from Dani, and let's start scratching the surface of how to break out of that box you're currently in!

Letter from Dani:

Why I created this book and started the Love Your Body mission.

With the impact of social media, we have become a world filled with edits, comparisons, and filters. My platform was built to support the idea that you can love yourself through movement and break the stereotype of what healthy and fit "have to look like." My goal is to help people become their best version, not a clone of someone else. Movement helps you feel strong, which leads to mental clarity, increased confidence, and a focus on your strengths instead of comparing yourself to everyone else.

By incorporating this idea into the fitness world and speaking/ teaching my clients, followers on social media, and even family members and friends, I have pioneered a way for people to start viewing a healthier relationship with exercise, food, and their bodies. Instead of sticking to the age-old mindset of waiting to love your body when you're "perfect" or at your "goal weight" to start being happy, I want people to start learning to love themselves now. I have found this approach to be a rarity in the fitness space. Letting go of expectations and deciding what I wanted to fight for is when I truly started loving myself and when I truly started living. I want this for everyone I work with, and I am here to help guide, support, and build the tools and structure to keep them healthy in mind, body, and spirit.

I want this brand to not just be recognized in Tennessee but all over the world someday as THE method and structure for helping you truly love yourself through My LYB Method, good movement, good fuel, and a positive mindset.

This road has never been easy. From the very start, my mottos and the idea of me being a female business owner in the fitness space, and even just a personal trainer, were always criticized and critiqued. I have continually proven my abilities over the years while dealing with verbal abuse, body shaming, discrimination, sexual misconduct, and not being taken seriously—whether it was due to my size, my age, or my gender. And going through these trials all while working towards creating my own real healthy lifestyle regimen.

My business started with the idea that there has to be intention in getting your movement in. Without a reason to "fight," why stick with it? My three mottos are: first, simply get your movement in (for longevity and health); second, fight for what YOU want (not what others want or society wants, but what you truly want); and lastly, the most important in my eyes: love your body throughout. Hating your way to "fit or skinny" is harmful and detrimental, and there's no space for that in my reality.

I have learned that it doesn't matter who doesn't support or see the vision; as long as you're clear, then you give it everything you have, and you will succeed. Maybe not in the way you thought and definitely not in the timeline you set for yourself, but if you keep going, you can overcome and become whatever you set your mind to.

I want the world, especially young women and girls reading this, to know you are not defined by your body and you do not have to stay within the box others have placed you in. You are more than a pretty face or a great body; you are fierce, adaptable, and creative. If you want to look your best, work hard to be your healthiest, one day at a time. If you want to be happy, stop waiting for an outside force to make you feel worthy, stop letting other people tell you who you are, and stop dimming your light.

You decide how you live this life. You have the freedom to choose, and I am here to support you in any way I can.

Love, Dani

My Personal Story with Hating My Body

After years in high school of feeling like the odd girl out, even into college, I continued listening to what others said about my body, and it dimmed my light. I had stopped looking at my body naked in the mirror, stopped dancing for a year, started drinking more, and wore baggier clothes. One day, in my junior year of college, when I was 20 years old, I had a realization that changed everything. I had decided to start getting my movement in a year prior, mainly running and teaching group fitness classes. Here I am now, getting paid in my second year of teaching and really embracing it and loving it, but something still felt like it was missing. I would stand in front of my computer and record while practicing my routines for my fitness format, which is now called MoveFit, in my apartment living room.

I would go back and watch to remember and build routines. I looked at a video after just recording, and I sat in disbelief that that was what I looked like. I didn't recognize myself. I then grabbed a calzone out of the fridge at 11 a.m. on a Tuesday and ate it as an emotional response to what I saw in that video.
After I ate the calzone, I said, "enough is enough. I have to start eating better because I love to move, and I want to help others do the same. I knew that I was great; I was meant to teach others, but I had to set an example and help myself first."
I started by giving up soda. Mind you, I used to drink 2 liters a day growing up, so this was a significant part of my life. I knew I couldn't have moderation with it, so cutting it out was a great start. The second thing I did was say no more fast food and started drinking alcohol less often.

This wasn't perfect eating or even weighing my food. I just started with these three things. Once I did this, I started to see slight changes in my body, had more energy, and felt a little better every day. All this to say, it's just like what you'll learn in this book. It's not just about whether you love yourself or you don't. You slowly start taking away a few of the negative comments you say daily, which will help tremendously. By doing so, it will free up space mentally for you to think of at least one positive thing. While I did this, I started taking pictures daily and slowly began feeling more comfortable in my body.

About a year after I started eating better and teaching group fitness classes, I started strength training, fell in love with it, and became a certified personal trainer. The confidence kept building from there. I started looking at myself in the mirror naked, something I couldn't do for years. I was so proud of myself that I could see my body and watch it change. I was finding one thing daily that I loved about it without the negatives always bringing me down. Even as silly as saying my eyelashes or my nails, I found one thing every day for years until it became second nature. Then I was able to just intuitively say what I loved and really mean it.

This is a process. Day by day, you will get there, but we have to start with the hard part first. Let's get to it.

The LYB Initiative

I started in 2022 going around asking people on Broadway in Nashville, "What do you love about your body?" This was uncomfortable at first. I set aside my insecurities about whether people would be mean or think it's silly and just went for it. I had a guy filming for me and another to help give out podcast stickers and info about my mission. Can you guess what most people said when asked this question? Most people told me what others have said they liked about their body, or that they didn't like anything. It was just as I had suspected. We live in a society where how could you love yourself if you're not the "societal standard"? It was a great day for research, stepping out of comfort zones, and I really enjoyed the interviewing process. From there, I posted clips all over social media showcasing this initiative. Fast forward to two years later, countless interviews from the Arnold Sports Festival in Ohio to New York Times Square, to the Music City Expo and interviewing the Olympian himself Jay Cutler. Every single interview where I ask at the end, "Has anyone ever asked you this question before?" Everyone's response is, "No, actually they haven't." THINK ABOUT THIS: think about how many times a day you talk negatively about your body to others and how no one has ever asked you what you love about your body. The response to negative comments is seen as normal, but what if we turned the negative into the positive? Imagine how different our conversations would be. I wanted to start asking others because I believe that when we ask this question, it opens up so many other questions. So that is where we will begin.

And I'll ask you...

CHAPTER 1: WHAT DO YOU LOVE ABOUT YOUR BODY?

Really take a second and ask yourself, "What do you love about your body?" This isn't about what others have told you they love, but deep down, what do you love? We first have to understand that the word "love" means: "an intense feeling of deep affection."

In today's society, we have held this word as such a taboo in conjunction with our own bodies. Why? Because you've been made to feel you're too much if you boast or are confident, or simply because society makes money off your insecurities and plays on them every moment of every day. Here's the latest cellulite cream, or expensive weight loss drug, or worse, they sell you that you can look like a Kardashian if you do X, Y, and Z.

Let's keep it real. I know what I am asking seems much harder, but how backwards is that? I do this "Love Your Body Initiative" where I ask people of all shapes, bodies, ages, and sizes what they love about their bodies. In every single interview, I ask, "Has anyone ever asked you this question?" You know what they say? They pause and say, "No, actually no one ever has." My response: "I am glad I could be the first."

This right here is why I wrote this guide: to help open up the dialogue of what, when, how, and why you can love your body throughout your journey. So let's get to it.

Your first LYB activity is below. On the provided lines, write what you love about your body, and beside it, write what you don't love about your body. If you can't think of anything, that's okay—you can focus on your strengths, your ability to have a child, or consider all the amazing things your body does for you.

What I Love about my body:

_____#_____

_____#_____

_____#_____

What I do not love about my body:

_____#_____

_____#_____

_____#_____

From here, I want you to write down the number of times you say the negative out loud or to yourself each day beside the comment.

Next, write down the same number beside what you said you love about your body.

Now, for each negative comment you wrote down, I want you to mark over the comment the number of times you wrote it down, literally blocking it out of your sight.

From here, focus only on the positive. Say out loud the description beside the positive comment that number of times.
Go ahead, no one's around. You've got this.

CHAPTER 2: WHY DON'T YOU LOVE YOUR BODY?

Identifying why you don't love your body:

Okay, so we've just completed your first LYB activity, and I'm incredibly proud of you! Did you notice how it might have felt a bit silly to repeat "I love my legs" 30 times, but how natural it is to criticize XYZ about your body to yourself, your friends, your partner, and loved ones every single day? It probably even felt awkward to compliment yourself that much—why is that?

Well, full disclosure: I'm not a therapist, but I do have a degree in Communications and have helped thousands with this very struggle, including myself. What I believe is that somewhere along the line, it became uncool to be confident because someone was always ready to shut down your positivity real quick. Maybe every time you got dressed for school or at school, you were compared to a classmate, friend, or sibling. Look, I'm not blaming anyone, but I truly understand how stressful, frustrating, and saddening it is to feel like you're lesser because you don't look a certain way. This is not a war against small bodies or large bodies; I want to make that very clear. You could have been made fun of for wearing glasses when others did not—something as simple as that.

I remember being called an ogre in 8th grade, one year after

I started public school. Trying to navigate that was really challenging. I genuinely didn't believe it until I put on weight due to medication, and then other comments came along, like being called a whale and being laughed at when I wore what I thought was cute by people who were my friends. I know how much these comments can stick with you, but they don't have to define you. What I came to realize was that I loved my body; it was others' words and comments that allowed them to steal my light and make me question if I should love it.

When I was 19 years old, I was at my heaviest and unhealthiest, feeling unhappy because I literally felt invisible to everyone, including myself in the mirror. I finally said, "Enough is enough," and told myself, regardless of my size, people will always find something to criticize. I am more than just my body, and now it's time to start fighting for what I want. For me, that meant feeling better and loving myself again. If you're like me and you need to start quieting the noise and stop seeking validation in others' opinions, here's your next step...

CHAPTER 3: WHEN DID YOU STOP LIKING YOUR BODY?

We have identified the what, and then why. Now, I encourage you to address when you started disliking your body, and after that, it's time to start retraining the way you view yourself.
Get a colorful sticky note of your favorite color.

Write on it what you love about your body. It can be as simple as your fingernails—just put something down.

Now, stick this on your mirror.

I want you to do this every day for the next 30 days and fill your mirror up. You can do anything for a month. It's important to do this consecutively, not just 30 days in general, as we are building real, long-lasting habits. If you skip or miss a day, I encourage you to start over. Trust me, it will be worth it. You got this!

CHAPTER 4: WHERE ARE YOU IN YOUR JOURNEY OF LOVING YOUR BODY?

I want you to circle on a scale of 1-10 how much you love your body.

Scale: 1 2 3 4 5 6 7 8 9 10

At the end of the 30 days of writing down either the same thing you love each day or something different on your sticky notes, I want you to come back here and see what number you circle now.

Scale: 1 2 3 4 5 6 7 8 9 10

If you see no change or notice the number go down, then I encourage you to continue with the sticky note method for another 30 days, persisting until your mindset begins to shift. If you feel you need more tools, I encourage you to revisit Activity 1. Write down all the things you hate about your body—not just one thing—and for each of those, say them aloud as you tear them up over a fire. Let them burn! This can be a powerful cleansing technique. There is more space for this activity in the back of the book titled "Light It Up!"

If you find yourself hating your body because of verbal abuse or body shaming, I understand. Here's the thing: at this point, it's about not believing the narratives from the prior trauma that your body can't be beautiful or seen as beautiful unless it looks a certain way. Here are a few things that help me feel good daily, which in turn help me love myself more:

Moving my body—movement has saved my life more times than I care to admit. It's a saving grace; when I feel mentally weak, I engage in a workout and come out stronger both mentally and physically. Movement won't fix your problems, but it will never talk back, question you, and it will be there to support you when you need it the most.

Fueling my body—I know, I know, you're like "Dani, pizza is life." I get it, and I do love it from time to time. But I also know how I feel when I don't nourish my body, especially as a woman with hormones and all the challenges that can arise. Prioritize lean protein, stay away from processed foods that give a dopamine high, and focus on steady, clean energy. This approach will help you feel and see a difference not just in weight, but in your skin, digestion, and healthier hair, etc. There's so much more to health than just weight loss.

Lastly, I believe in the power of manifestation. If you believe you attract positive things, then you will. If you tell yourself every day how unattractive or sad you are, then you will embody that. The beauty of this life is that YOU decide how you wish to see yourself. And I believe with my LYB Method you can change your perspective by living out a real, healthy lifestyle regimen.

CHAPTER 5: HOW TO STAY ON YOUR JOURNEY OF LOVING YOUR BODY THROUGHOUT.

It's not easy; people will tear you down, doubt you—yes, even people you love. But that's the beauty of this whole topic. It's not about how to get others to love your body or how to fit into someone else's idea of perfection. It's about how to stay on YOUR journey of loving YOUR body throughout.

-Quiet the noise around you and avoid comparisons.

-Start moving your body—whether through going on walks or strength training; both are great starts.

-Work on your affirmations daily.

-Engage in the Love Your Body activities I've shared with you.

-Establish a routine with these practices, and you will never look back.

Take it step by step, day by day, and know that you can love yourself throughout. If you need more help in doing so, I would love to work with you one-on-one for coaching, training, or have you join any of my quarterly challenges. I understand this all may feel like a lot to ask, but it's no different than starting a new job, a new workout regimen, or dating someone new. There's fear around all those things, but once you're in it, you learn so much about yourself, and that's what loving your body throughout is all about.

I believe it's key in your success to love your body and yourself that you have things around you or that you wear that motivate or inspire you daily. Here's your last activity!

Activity: Create Your LYB Vision Board

Purpose: To visualize and manifest your goals for self-love and body-positive fitness.

Instructions:
Gather Materials: You'll need a poster board or a large piece of paper, magazines, scissors, glue, and markers. If you prefer, you can create a digital version using apps like Canva.

Reflect: Take a moment to think about what LYB means to you. Consider how you want to feel about your body and what specific goals you want to achieve on your journey without comparison.

Collect Images and Words: Flip through magazines and cut out images, quotes, and words that resonate with your vision of self-love, empowerment, and confidence.

Assemble Your Board: Arrange the images and words on your board in a way that feels good to you. There's no right or wrong way to do this! Glue everything down, and don't forget to add your personal touches with markers—write affirmations or goals directly on the board.

Display Your Board: Find a prominent place to hang your vision board where you'll see it daily. This will serve as a constant reminder of your commitment to loving your body and the goals you've set for yourself.

Reflect Regularly: Spend a few minutes each week reflecting on your vision board. Are you making progress toward your goals? What feelings does it evoke? Update it as needed to reflect your evolving journey.

Once you've created your LYB Vision Board, consider sharing it with friends or on social media. Tag me! @danidfitness1 - Would love to connect with you on your LYB journey!

As you embark on this journey, remember that loving your body is a continuous process that requires patience, dedication, and self-compassion. Embrace the small victories, celebrate your progress, and be kind to yourself along the way. You have the power to redefine what it means to be healthy and happy in your own skin. Thank you for allowing me to be a part of your journey. Let's keep moving forward together, one step at a time. Time to change the situation!

INSPIRATION
What do you love about your body?

What I love about my body is the newfound freedom and love I feel for it. When I first started working with Dani, I struggled with negative thoughts and couldn't imagine loving myself. However, through Dani's individual and intentional approach, I've experienced a complete mindset shift. As Katie said, "The consequences of revamping my mindset equal a change in my perspective, leading to physical changes and ultimately a freedom and love for my body that I never thought possible." Now, I find joy in my reflection and pride in my progress, grateful every day for Dani's belief in me and her help in fighting for what I wanted—learning to love my body.

-Katie

What I love about my body is the appreciation and love I've learned to have for it, thanks to Dani D Fitness. When I started with Dani D in 2021, her passion and dedication made me feel welcomed and appreciated. She taught me to cherish my health and body like never before. As one client shared, "During that time, she taught me how to love my body and appreciate my health more than ever before." Dani D and her community have inspired me to fight for what I want and embrace self-love and care. Her impact on my life is something I will always cherish.

-Ashley

What I love about my body are my quads—my "thickkk thighs" that never let me down in a workout. Dani D Fitness has taught me to focus on what I am proud of rather than getting stuck on things I wish would change. As Heather said, "There's always something to love about your body; and it's through DDF challenges that I've focused on what I am proud of." Dani's support for all body types and performance levels has helped me appreciate and celebrate my body's strengths.

-Heather

What I love about my body is the resilience and strength I've discovered through working with Dani D. Fitness. Meeting Dani at the Nashville Fit Expo in 2023, I was struggling with chronic health issues and felt like I'd lost my shine. However, Dani's mission to "Love Your Body" helped me see past what my body couldn't do and focus on what it could. As one client shared, "Thank you Dani for helping me see myself in a new light, so that I can keep fighting for what I want!" Despite setbacks, I've learned to appreciate my body's capabilities and celebrate its strength and beauty every day.

-Mary

What I love about my body is the confidence I've gained to embrace and celebrate it. After a few years of training with Dani D. Fitness and seeing her openness about her own journey, I finally wore a two-piece bikini in public. As one client shared, "Dani has taught me to be kind to myself and to focus on the positive changes in my body." While I'm still learning to love certain aspects of my body, the biggest milestone has been realizing that I'm living a healthy lifestyle and embracing my body without fear of judgment. Dani's guidance has helped me focus on positivity and self-kindness.

-Wendy

What I love about my body is the strength and capability of my legs. After training with Dani D. Fitness, I learned to prioritize my health and appreciate what my body can do. As one client shared, "Right now, I am LOVING my legs and what they can do for me. This summer, my husband and I have been to the beach, the College World Series, gone on hikes, and moved some HEAVY furniture and my legs have been healthy and strong for me!" Dani's support and the Love Your Body community have taught me to love my body throughout all phases of life, knowing that I am capable, strong, and giving my body what it needs to be the best version of myself.

-Chelsey

What I love about my body is the strength and capability of my legs. Through Dani's programming focused on being strong and loving your body, I've gained a total appreciation for what my body can do rather than just how it looks. As one client shared, "What I love most about my body currently are my legs—they never fail me when walking around my city, mowing my lawn, or carrying heavy objects. I love how muscular they are!" This perspective shift has helped me love and appreciate my body's strength and functionality.

-Andrea

What I love about my body is the strength of my legs. Dani has taught me to truly appreciate and love my body for what it can do. As one client shared, "I, as a 47-year-old female, have never felt so healthy and strong. The one thing that I am proud of is my strong legs!" Dani's perspective on body positivity has inspired my family and me to lead a healthy lifestyle and be positive role models for our daughter. Our bodies may not look like "model" types, but we are moving daily and being the healthiest individuals we can be. Thanks to Dani, we've embraced a mindset that "everybody matters" and learned to love our bodies in all seasons.

-Mandy

What I love about my body is the strength and resilience of my legs. Working with Dani D. Fitness has shown me the importance of daily movement and its profound impact on mental health. As one client shared, "A morning walk has become my reset or 'Happiness Trigger.'" This routine has helped me feel stronger and more connected to my mind and body, especially as I navigate perimenopause at 52. Dani and her community of strong women have been instrumental in my journey towards better health and wellness. Through their support, I've found more positivity in life and feel confident in showing my body in public.

-Allison

What I love about my body is its strength and resilience, thanks to working out with Dani. Battling body dysmorphia and disordered eating since I was 12, I used to strive for my smallest self. Now, with DDF, I strive to be my strongest, healthiest self. As ME shared, Dani's guidance has given me a new appreciation for what my body is capable of.

-M.E.

The LYB mission to me means loving yourself and your body through all seasons. Not only loving yourself aesthetically but mentally as well. Every day consciously make the choice to love yourself and that includes loving your body. You have to be able to give yourself grace. Not every day is going to be the best day and that's okay! The most important thing is to never give up on yourself because you deserve the best you have to give.

-Amanda

LIGHT IT UP

The "Light It Up!" section is designed to provide additional space for you to engage in the powerful cleansing activity described earlier. Use these pages to write down all the negative thoughts you have about your body. When you're ready, follow the steps to safely burn these notes, symbolizing the release of negativity and the creation of space for a more positive mindset. Remember, this is a continuous journey, and these extra pages are here to support you whenever you need them.

_____

_____

_____

_____

_____

_____

_____

_____

_____

_____

_____

_____

_____

_____

_____

_____

_____

_____

_____

_____

_____

_____

_____

_____

_____

_____

_____

_____

_____   Love Your Body.

Email: dani@danidfitness.com

For more information, visit our website at danidfitness.com

Disclaimer: This book is for informational purposes only and is intended to help guide you on your journey to a healthier life through movement. Dani D. Fitness is not a licensed therapist; she is a holistic health coach with 12 years of experience as a certified group fitness instructor and personal trainer. She has also run a successful business since 2017 and has gone through this journey just like you. This book is meant to be a tool, not the ultimate solution for your relationship with your body and mind. My hope and goal are that you will start loving yourself more each day.

ABOUT THE AUTHOR

Danielle Dyer

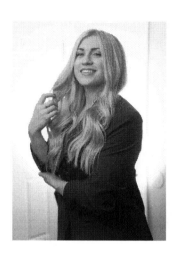

DANIELLE DYER, OWNER OF DANI D. FITNESS, IS A CERTIFIED HEALTH AND FITNESS PROFESSIONAL, SPEAKER, HOST OF "THE LOVE YOUR BODY" PODCAST, CREATOR OF THE BODY-POSITIVE FITNESS FORMAT MOVEFIT, AUTHOR, AND FOLLOWER OF CHRIST.

Made in the USA
Columbia, SC
21 October 2024

44459835R00024